crisisnotes

crisisnotes

Practical Suggestions for Living Through a
Challenging Experience

MARK D. LERNER, PH.D.

MARK LERNER ASSOCIATES, INC.
NEW YORK

Published by Mark Lerner Associates, Inc.

crisisnotes

© 2012 by Mark D. Lerner, Ph.D.

The suggestions in this book are intended solely for informational and educational purposes and not as medical or psychological advice. If you have questions or concerns regarding your health, please consult with your healthcare provider.

FIRST EDITION

Mark Lerner Associates, Inc. Publications
P.O. Box 1315
Melville, N.Y. 11747

crisisnotes.com

Tel. (631) 673-3513

Library of Congress Control Number: 2012901462
ISBN 978-0-9772818-3-1

Although we cannot change our circumstance,
we can choose how we respond to it.

INTRODUCTION

cri·sis /ˈkrīsis/ noun, plural -ses

1. A crucial or decisive point or situation;
    a turning point.
2. An emotionally stressful event or traumatic
    change in a person's life.

This book was inspired by my clients and friends—people who have turned to me for over twenty-five years for help during life's most challenging times.

The question I frequently hear during a crisis is, "What can I do now?"

Crisisnotes will guide you from the earliest phase of your experience through the healing process. Because the challenges we face are so diverse, consider those suggestions that are appropriate to your circumstance. And certainly, add your own notes in the space provided.

So many people have utilized the contents of this book to move from victim to survivor and, ultimately, thriver. Let *crisisnotes* provide the timely information, inspiration and hope that you need now.

Address your medical needs first. If at any time you are having difficulty breathing, or experiencing chest pains or palpitations, seek immediate medical attention.

1

Surround yourself with
your family and loved ones.

2

Talk about what's happened, tell your story
and allow yourself to feel.

3

Drink plenty of water.

4

Make your physical safety and
well-being a priority.

5

Try to obtain the facts concerning
what has happened.

6

Allow trusted family members or friends to
help you make important decisions.

7

Spend time with people
who listen more than they speak.

8

Have tissues available.

9

See your reactions as normal responses
to an abnormal event.

10

Know that your feelings are
not right or wrong; they just are.

11

Avoid withdrawing.

12

Let yourself cry with a friend.

13

Know that it's common for things to seem surreal,
as if you're watching yourself in a movie.

14

Consider how your experience is
affecting you spiritually.

15

If you feel so inclined, pray.

16

$\mathcal{D}$on't be afraid to ask for help.

17

$\mathcal{N}$ever apologize for showing your feelings.

18

$\mathcal{R}$ealize that repetitive recollections of
what happened are normal.

19

$\mathcal{A}$void sharing strong feelings in text messages.

20

Know that sleep problems are among the
most common reactions during a crisis.

21

Eliminate caffeine for four hours prior to bedtime.

22

Understand that nightmares are very common.

23

*F*ocus on the here and now, and
live in the present moment.

24

*W*hen you're feeling overwhelmed,
take a slow deep breath, inhaling through
your nose, hold your breath for five seconds
and then exhale slowly through your mouth.
Upon exhalation, think the word "relax."
Repeat this process several times.

25

Realize that headaches and
an upset stomach are common.

26

Take care of your personal hygiene.

27

Know that you may feel numb.

28

If you find it difficult to concentrate when
someone is speaking to you, focus on
the specific words being said and
slow down the conversation.

29

Know that you are the expert in being you.
No one has the right to tell you
how you should feel.

30

Spend time with children.

31

Encourage children to share
their feelings with you.

32

Assure children that they are safe.

33

If you don't know the answer to a child's question,
tell her that you don't know.

34

*R*ecognize that children often
regress during a crisis.

35

*T*ell children the truth, at a
developmentally appropriate level.

36

*H*elp adolescents to maintain
positive peer relationships.

37

Know that familiar habits and routines
can provide comfort.

38

Resist the urge to shut down.

39

Accept help.

40

Understand that it's common
to be easily frustrated.

41

Survive one hour at a time and,
eventually, one day at a time.

42

Realize that your experience may
compromise your ability to think clearly.

43

Know that it's common to have
difficulty sitting still.

44
Recognize that your experience is likely
affecting your family and friends.

45
Know that a loss of appetite is common.

46
Eat small, healthy snacks.

47
Have a family meeting to foster communication.

48

*K*now that feelings of loneliness are
very common and normal.

49

*B*ecome aware of and slow down your breathing.

50

*T*ake a long, hot shower.

51

*U*nderstand that you are not
"losing it" or "going crazy."

52

If you find it difficult to concentrate when someone is speaking to you, try repeating what you have just heard.

53

Excuse yourself from people who lecture you.

54

When appropriate, attend a funeral or memorial service.

55

Grieve freely.

56

Know that it's okay not to be okay, right now.

57

Consider that there may be "hidden victims"—
others who have been impacted by your experience.

58

Avoid increased tobacco use.

59

Know that your experience may rekindle
recollections of earlier traumatic events in your life.

60

Know that normal people often
feel abnormal when faced with a crisis.

61

Make a list of priorities.

62

Accept support.

63

Don't fight your feelings.

64

Know that many people
question their faith.

65

Go to your house of worship.

66

Speak with your spiritual leader.

67

*R*esist the urge to retreat into your own world.

68

*R*ecognize that crying is a
natural tension-release mechanism.

69

*K*now that yearning and searching are common
among people who have experienced a loss.

70

Speak with your physician or
healthcare provider about what has happened.

71

Get three medical opinions when faced with
a serious health problem.

72

*I*f you don't feel safe with yourself, speak with a family member and your healthcare provider.

73

*D*on't make a promise you can't keep.

74

*C*reate a diary or journal.

75

Know that you are not your body. While your
body may be broken, it does not mean that you are.

76

Avoid impulsive, emotional decisions.

77

Avoid advice-givers.

78

*D*o one thing at a time.

79

*W*hen making decisions, try to keep yourself in thinking rather than feeling mode.

80

Don't allow anyone to talk you into something
that makes you feel uncomfortable.

81

Understand that being easily startled and
feeling jumpy is very common.

82

Know that your emotional pain
will ease with time.

83

*P*roblem-solve with your friends.

84

*A*sk family and friends to check-in with you.

85

*S*ay "no" to things you don't want to do.

86

Know that it's not unusual to feel the presence of someone who has died.

87

Avoid alcohol as a sleep aid.

88

Resist emailing when you're emotionally consumed.

89

*U*nderstand that feelings of emptiness are normal.

90

*R*ecognize that what you think
will affect the way you feel.

91

*C*ommunicate facts and dispel rumors.

92

*A*pologize when appropriate.

93

Know that others may say things
to try to help you to feel better quickly.
They may need to feel better quickly.

94

Face your feelings.

95

Avoid avoidance.

96

Draw upon past experiences to
help you to cope today.

97

Limit the amount of exposure to
your story if it's on television.

98

Take your regular medications.

99

Know that loud noises may easily startle you.

100

Give yourself "reality checks."
Focus on the facts and see things as they are.

101

*K*now that "man-made" tragedies
often hurt the most.

102

*T*alk about feelings of sadness and depression.

103

Speak with a counselor or therapist.

104

Express your feelings of frustration and anger.

105

Know that panic attacks are among
the most common reasons people
turn to professionals for help.

106

When you are feeling angry, pause,
then slowly count to ten.

107

Know that you will likely ride
an emotional roller coaster.

108

Appreciate that you may feel worse
before you begin to feel better.

109

Remind yourself that you will get through this.

110

Set limits and boundaries
when dealing with others.

111

Speak with your healthcare provider if
an inability to sleep continues to be a problem.

112

Understand that during peak emotional
experiences, what you think about and
focus on will stay with you.

113

Speak with a professional if you are troubled with
"flashbacks"—feeling as if you are reliving the
event over and over again.

114

Know that there are many ways to cope.
One approach, or strategy, doesn't fit all.

115

When appropriate, consult with an attorney.

116

If necessary, have a spokesperson.

117

If you must make a statement to the press,
focus on those who were adversely impacted.

118

Clarify published inaccuracies early on.

119

Understand that you will likely remember
whatever you do during a peak
emotional experience.

120

Have alone time with your spouse or partner.

121

Read a story to a child.

122

Focus on what really matters.

123

Play soft, relaxing background music.

124

Learn to distract yourself.

125

Understand that physical injury and pain
increases the likelihood of emotional pain.

126

To relax, focus on the movement
of the clouds.

127

Consider speaking with a psychiatrist
about medications that can help you.

128

Ask your healthcare provider whether
a sleep aid may help you to sleep.

129

Do one thing at a time.

130

*K*now that while you can't change
what's happened, you can choose
how you will respond to it.

131

*T*urn to a pediatrician with
questions about children.

132

*T*urn to your family with financial concerns.

133

Recognize how your experience is
affecting your thoughts.

134

Let others know that you need
to talk and "vent."

135

Be aware of how you are displacing
your feelings of anger.

136

*I*dentify the connection between
your thoughts and your feelings.

137

*B*ecome aware of thoughts
that make your symptoms worse.

138

If you have chest pains,
speak with your healthcare provider, now.

139

Try to remain calm and patient.

140

Don't blame yourself.

141

Ask yourself, "Who else may be hurting?"

142

Learn to identify your anxiety triggers.

143

Try to stop self-defeating thoughts early.
Catch yourself and say, "This is not productive."

144

*O*pen windows and let in fresh air.

145

*A*void alcohol and drugs.

146

*B*e realistic.

147

*G*ive yourself permission to rest.

148

When necessary, go with a family member
or friend to the doctor.

149

Don't make major decisions quickly.

150

Don't over-schedule.

151

Avoid bickering and fighting.

152

*E*xcuse yourself when people speak of others who have had the same experience.

153

*A*void people who have all the answers.

154

*F*ind the right people with whom to speak.

155

Listen to your inner voice.

156

Reflect on good memories.

157

Have alone time with your children.

158

When feeling emotionally overwhelmed,
change what you are doing.

159

Recognize that during a crisis you will lose a sense of control. You can regain control by focusing on what you can do now.

160

Don't become consumed with reading about your story if it's online or in the newspaper.

161

*R*ealize that you are not your crisis.

162

*H*elp others to know
how they can support you.

163

*D*on't be critical of yourself or others.

164

Communicate with your co-workers.

165

When appropriate, consult with a
Human Resources representative.

166

Keep employees informed.

167

Know that people remember
what a leader does during a crisis.

168

Know that people often become leaders
because of what they do during a crisis.

169

Consider hiring a crisis management consultant.

170

Beware of increased suggestibility.
You may be easily influenced.

171

Learn more about your healthcare providers.

172

Visualize a relaxing place.

173

When appropriate, communicate with your children's teachers and school administrators.

174

Cut back on commitments.

175

Focus on what you can do.

176

If you can, postpone major decisions.

177

When appropriate, speak with
your insurance company.

178

Get estimates.

179

Keep receipts.

180

When appropriate,
photograph injuries or damage.

181

Don't give away original documents.

182

Pay your bills.

183

Establish a budget.

184

When appropriate, consult with an accountant.

185

*K*now that you wont "get over it."
You will learn to get through it.

186

*B*eware of negative self-talk.

187

*U*se positive coping statements such as,
"I am going to overcome this."

188

Know that how you label your experience
will affect how you feel about it.

189

Remain sensitive to cultural differences in
how people respond during a crisis.

190
Create the best sleep environment you can.

191
Use a night light if it's helpful.

192
Consider using a sound conditioning machine
to help you sleep.

193

Consider family counseling.

194

Write a letter expressing your feelings.

195

Listen to your favorite music.

196

Avoid people who have all the answers.

197

Strive to be your best.

198

Take a warm bath.

199
Switch from thinking to doing.

200
Turn off your cell phone.

201
Choose your focus.

202
Create a schedule.

203

Educate yourself about your symptoms.

204

Know that knowledge is power.

205

Spend time with positive people.

206

Read inspirational quotes.

207

*K*now that feeling angry is normal,
but be aware of how you express your anger.

208

*L*earn to stop and pause when
you're feeling frustrated or angry.

209

*U*se relaxation techniques.

210
Take vitamins.

211
Get out in daylight.

212
Wear clothing that helps you to feel better.

213
Do what feels right for you.

214

Avoid labeling yourself with a disorder.

215

Don't be impulsive.

216

Avoid negative people.

217

Don't blame others.

218

Light a fire in a fireplace
and turn on soft music.

219

Let someone babysit.

220

Listen to your body and take naps.

221

Know that feelings of guilt are very common.

222

Decide when it's really worth getting upset.

223

Close your eyes and
envision yourself at the beach.

224

Simplify your life.

225

*K*now that children, particularly little ones,
will take their cues from the adults
around them during a crisis.

226

*E*nlist the help of a child psychologist to
address specific questions you may have.

227

If you've been harmed,
have the benefit of legal counsel.

228

Know that physical discomfort can
serve as a trigger for emotional discomfort.

229

See physical pain as a signal to
speak with your healthcare provider.

230

See disturbing dreams as your mind working overtime, trying to make sense of the senseless.

231

Eat a healthy diet.

232

Try to be brave.

233

*K*now that being excessively
watchful and cautious is normal.

234

*B*eware of the impact of your crisis on others.

235

*T*ake short breaks.

236
*W*rite a poem.

237
*T*ry muscle relaxation techniques.
Tighten and loosen your muscles from
the top of your head to the tips of your toes.

238

Notice that children often communicate
their feelings through their actions.

239

Encourage children to share their
thoughts and feelings using their words.

240

Consider removing unhealthy reminders
from your home.

241

Work to get "unstuck."

242

Listen to music from a happy time in your life.

243

Sketch a drawing of whatever comes to mind.

244

Understand that knowledge
will give you back a sense of control.

245

Turn to experts.

246

Recognize that "survivor guilt" is common.

247

Read and learn about traumatic stress.

248

*U*nderstand that one approach
will not help everyone. You are unique.

249

*C*onsider marital counseling.

250

*H*ave a massage.

251

*T*ry reflexology.

252

Embrace your faith.

253

Read the bible.

254

Connect with nature.

255

Give yourself permission to relax.

256
Have coffee with a friend.

257
Become more active.

258
Make goal-directed decisions.

259
Avoid procrastinating.

260
Take a brisk walk.

261
Go for a run.

262
Work out.

263
Eat a balanced diet.

264

*P*icture yourself at a special place.

265

*D*o something you enjoy.

266

*I*nstead of focusing on the problem,
focus on the solution.

267

Recognize the power of your choices.

268

Join a support group.

269

Beware of black and white,
"all good or all bad," thinking.

270

Work to channel your energy
in a positive direction.

271

Write down three things
for which you are grateful.

272

Learn to forgive yourself.

273

*U*nderstand that a crisis is in the eye of the beholder. What is a crisis for you may not be for someone else ... and vice versa.

274

*K*now that some people refer to a "new normal" after experiencing a traumatic event.

275

Reflect on an achievement you have made.

276

Realize that while time doesn't
heal all wounds, it does give us the
opportunity to learn how we can cope.

277

Accept that pain and disappointment
are a part of life.

278

Write down your thoughts
before going to bed.

279

Read a new book.

280

Listen to an audiobook.

281

Know that healing is a journey.

282

*R*ecognize that countless people
live through adversity.

283

*G*radually expose yourself to your fears.

284

*T*ake responsibility for your mistakes.

285

Focus on the facts,
rather than "what ifs."

286

Seek out experts online.

287

Accept that life isn't fair.

288

Notice how your experience
is affecting your actions.

289

Recognize that what you focus on
becomes your experience.

290

Recognize that blaming others doesn't help.

291

As you have a painful thought,
label it as unproductive and dismiss it.

292

Strive to be the way you
would ideally like to see yourself.

293

If you're having suicidal thoughts,
share them with your physician or
healthcare provider now.

294

Use your pain as fuel to overcome your crisis.

295

Consider that we only see a rainbow
after the rain.

296

*R*ecognize the power of your decisions.

297

*M*ake decisions based upon pros and cons.

298

*S*chedule a physical examination.

299

*B*ecome aware of your posture.

300

Trust your instincts.

301

Be careful not to burn bridges.

302

Speak with someone who has
experienced a similar event.

303

Become involved in an
online discussion forum.

304

Use your experience as a powerful lesson
for the children in your life.

305

Spend time with people who
help you to feel better.

306

Rekindle an old friendship.

307

Adjust your work schedule.

308

Take mental health days.

309

Identify one thing you can do each day
that makes you feel good.

310

*U*nderstand that facing adversity
is a part of life.

311

*G*ive yourself time to heal.

312

*R*ecognize how your experience is
affecting you, physically.

313

Consider biofeedback.

314

Consider seeing a chiropractor.

315

Try aromatherapy.

316

Consider using herbal remedies and oils.

317

Consider acupuncture.

318

Consider music and art therapies.

319

Keep up with local and world news.

320

*L*earn that you have the answers inside you.

321

*R*eflect on something you did well as a child.

322

*R*ecall fond memories.

323

*S*urround yourself with
photographs of good times.

324
Have the courage to move ahead.

325
Decide to let go.

326
Make informed, healthy,
goal-directed choices.

327
Never, ever, give up!

328
*W*rite a letter.

329
*R*ead an inspirational book.

330
*N*otice how your real friends stick by you.

331

*A*sk yourself, "What can I do?"—
instead of focusing on what you can't.

332

*K*now that while challenges don't define us,
how we respond to them often does.

333
*I*dentify your fears.

334
*E*xpose yourself to what frightens you.

335
*D*o something you always wanted to do.

336

*M*editate with positive affirmations
such as "I grow from this experience."

337

*E*xperience hypnosis and learn self-hypnosis.

338

*L*isten to a motivational lecture.

339

Thank someone who inspires you.

340

Choose to persevere.

341

Identify a quality you admire about yourself.

342

*M*ake a list of what helps you to feel better.

343

*B*ecome more flexible.

344

*R*ecognize that humor can help.

345
Keep exercising.

346
Read about inspirational people
who have overcome adversity.

347
Identify something that makes you unique.

348

Know that you have the power to
overcome your challenge.

349

Cultivate a mission and a
new sense of purpose.

350

Start a blog.

351

*R*ealize that you are not your past.

352

*L*earn to forgive others.

353

*B*ecome a better listener.

354

*D*iscuss these notes with your family,
friends and support group.

355

*F*ocus on what you want.

356

*V*isualize the attainment of a specific goal.

357

*M*ake deals with yourself to accomplish goals.

358

*R*ecognize that adversity can be a lesson.

359

*T*ake time to "recharge your battery."

360

*S*ee crises as opportunities.

361

*R*ead a biography of someone
who has overcome a challenge.

362

*R*emind yourself that there are others
who have faced a similar experience.

263

*W*atch family videos.

364

*L*ook at a photo album.

365

*C*reate a collage.

366

Make a list of options.

367

Find a mentor.

368

Consider enlisting the help of a life coach.

369

See a nutritionist.

370

Hire a personal trainer.

371

Lose weight.

372

$\mathcal{F}$ocus on where you wish to go,
rather than where you have been.

373

$\mathcal{B}$ecome your own best friend.

374

$\mathcal{B}$ecome more empathic in dealing with others.
Try to convey an understanding of the feelings
behind peoples' words.

375
Take a vacation.

376
Finish this sentence,
"If I could do anything, I would...."

377
Install a bird feeder and watch for guests.

378

*K*now that anniversaries and holidays
will be difficult.

379

*R*ecognize that we don't grow when we are
comfortable. We grow when we are challenged.

380

*W*rite down several short-term,
middle-term and long-term goals.

381

*D*o something that you enjoyed as a teenager.

382

*T*reasure your memories.

383

Learn never to leave a crisis without
looking for an opportunity to grow.

384

Imagine how you would like to
see yourself at this time next year.

385

Shift your focus from the problem
to the solution.

386

Strive to become more patient.

387

Be optimistic.

388

Be realistic.

389
See yourself moving from
victim to survivor and, ultimately, thriver.

390
Work to become the person
you would ideally like to be.

391
See your crisis as an opportunity for
self-improvement.

392

See overcoming your challenge as a journey.

393

Begin to write your autobiography.

394

Learn to let go.

395

Know that for many people,
acceptance is key.

396

Become more assertive.

397

Seek new role models.

398

Focus on growing from your experience
rather than bouncing back.

399
Help someone who is hurting.

400
Volunteer for a cause.

401
Visit a disabled or elderly person.

402
Donate to your favorite charity.

403

Start a charity.

404

Start a foundation.

405

Hold a fundraiser.

406

Write down a list of five things
you would like to do.

407

Think about what makes you happy.

408

Reflect on your successes.

409

Involve yourself in a cause.

410

Write a letter to the editor of a newspaper.

411

*H*elp someone who is facing a challenge.

412

*M*ake the best of your life.
It's the only one you will have.

413

*B*ecome more accepting.

414

Set goals, make decisions and take action.

415

Pursue your passion.

416

Choose to thrive.

417

Surround yourself with happy people.

418

Join a club.

419

Make each moment count.

420

Take a walk every morning.

421

Discover what makes you truly happy.

422

Start living your dreams.

423

Find a new hobby.

424

*U*se your strengths.

425

*S*peak to a group of young people
about your experience.

426

*G*o on a spontaneous trip.

427
Record a podcast.

428
Write a play.

429
Compose a song.

430
Play a musical instrument.

431

Volunteer in a homeless shelter.

432

Donate blood.

433

*W*rite a letter to someone who has
helped to change your life.

434

*B*ecome more positive and enthusiastic.

435

Take an adult education course.

436

Join your local fire department
or rescue squad.

437

Become an expert on something.

438

Wake up early and write.

439

Help someone achieve a goal.

440

Be there for someone
who is living through a crisis.

441

Do something for someone, anonymously.

442

*W*rite a story about overcoming adversity.

443

*W*rite an article.

444

*S*tart an online radio program.

445

Become your own hero.

446

Keep envisioning yourself the way
you would ideally like to be.

447

Volunteer in a hospital or nursing home.

448

Volunteer in a soup kitchen.

449

Make a donation to a college or university.

450

Present your story in your house of worship
or at your neighborhood library.

451

Establish new connections online.

452

Visit CrisisNotes.com.

453

*T*ell yourself,
"If it is to be, it is up to me."

454

*R*un for public office.

455

*S*tart your own business.

456

*W*rite your memoirs.

457
Inspire others.

458
Become a motivational speaker.

459
Travel the world.

460

Write a book about your experience.

461

Identify what has helped you the most.

462

Update your resume.

463

Explore a new career path.

464

*T*each a course.

465

*C*elebrate your accomplishments.

466

*B*e there for others.

467

*K*now that the answer to what you
ultimately need to do lies within you.

For more information about Dr. Mark Lerner and *crisisnotes*, please visit **CrisisNotes.com** or telephone (631) 673-3513.